This journal belongs to:

_____

Disclaimer

All information and resources found in this book are based on the opinions of the author, Michele Spring. Please consult your doctor before making any healthcare decisions. Michele Spring is not a doctor, lawyer, psychiatrist, nor therapist and no part of this book shall be interpreted as a diagnosis for any medical condition. The information in this book is not intended to replace a relationship with a qualified healthcare professional and is not intended as medical advice.

Copyright

ISBN-13: 978-1720238638

For more, visit thrivingonpaleo.com

Introduction

In 2014 my life completely changed. I'd been suffering from extreme exhaustion each day from 2pm until I went to bed, and then either I'd sleep for 14 hours and wake up just as tired or I'd have insomnia all night.

I had other symptoms too, like I was constantly cold, my hair was falling out, I had dry skin, I couldn't lose the baby weight, I had anxiety, constant brain fog was normal, and so much more.

My doctor had diagnosed me with hypothyroidism 8 years prior to this, but despite being on medication, I still wasn't feeling better.

2014 was the year I couldn't take it anymore. I was watching my life go by without living. My kids had that look - you know, the one where they're disappointed that you rejected them, AGAIN. It wasn't by choice. I just didn't have the energy to play with them, no matter how much I wanted to.

That year I found out I had not one, but two autoimmune diseases (Hashimoto's Thyroiditis and Celiac Disease) and that I could use diet and lifestyle changes to feel better.

And man, did I feel better once I did this. I went from what I described above to feeling absolutely FANTASTIC. Better than I'd felt in over 15 years.

How did I do it? I used the Paleo diet and subsets like Autoimmune Paleo (AIP) and Whole30 to stop the inflammation, settle my immune system down, and put my diseases into remission.

I talk all about this over on my blog and vlog at thrivingonpaleo.com, so if you're interested in learning more, come join me.

In the meantime though, this journal is the exact one I use any time I feel like I need to track how I'm doing.

How to use this journal

This journal has several places to track your progress as the 30 days goes on. You'll start first with an overview of your main goals and symptoms. Then you'll move into daily tracking of your food, sleep quality and hours, any movement/exercise throughout the day, energy and stress levels, and any symptoms and notes for the day.

This isn't meant to be a weight loss journal, nor does it really track macros or calories. Instead it aims to track symptoms and how you feel.

Use this as more of a guide that shows your own personal roadmap of foods that might be triggers for your symptoms. Took gluten out for 24 days and then had it on day 25, and you suddenly looked pregnant and couldn't remember your own name? Gluten might be an issue for you...

If you're doing a specific 30-day effort, you might notice that in the beginning you have a lot of symptoms, and then as you near day 30, many of those are gone. Celebrate this! This journal makes that easy since you can go back and see what you were suffering from in the beginning.

You can track your food however you want, but I recommend just giving a general idea, for example, "Tuna salad with mayo (tuna, celery, walnut, cranberries, mustard seed, Primal Kitchen Mayo)." I find tracking more than that cumbersome and tiring, but if you want to track things like carbs or calories, by all means, go for it.

Make sure to pay attention to things like your sleep, stress, and movement too as food doesn't paint the whole picture. These lifestyle components are also critical to feeling your best, and without dialing those in you'll most likely continue to feel subpar.

Ready to start?

WEEK 1

Main goals for the 30 days:

Symptoms I'm currently experiencing:

Goals for the coming week:

Day 1
Week 1

Date [   ]

_____

Breakfast: _____
_____
_____

Lunch: _____
_____
_____

Dinner: _____
_____
_____

Snacks: _____
_____

Sleep: QUALITY: ☺   😐   ☹

HOURS: 4 5 6 7 8 9 10

COMMENTS: _____
_____

Movement/Exercise: _____
_____
_____

Energy Level: 1 2 3 4 5 6 7 8 9 10

Stress Level: 1 2 3 4 5 6 7 8 9 10

Notes: (Cravings, Major Breakthroughs, Tough Spots, Symptoms):
_____
_____
_____
_____

"Every journey begins with a single step" - Maya Angelou

Day 2
Week 1

Date _____

Breakfast: _____
_____
_____

Lunch: _____
_____
_____

Dinner: _____
_____
_____

Snacks: _____
_____

Sleep:
HOURS: 4 5 6 7 8 9 10   QUALITY: 🙂   😐   🙁

COMMENTS: _____
_____

Movement/Exercise: _____
_____
_____

Energy Level: 1 2 3 4 5 6 7 8 9 10

Stress Level: 1 2 3 4 5 6 7 8 9 10

Notes: (Cravings, Major Breakthroughs, Tough Spots, Symptoms):
_____
_____
_____
_____
_____

"Strive for progress, not perfection"

Day 3
Week 1

Date

Breakfast: _____
_____

Lunch: _____
_____

Dinner: _____
_____

Snacks: _____

Sleep: QUALITY: ☺   😐   ☹
HOURS: 4 5 6 7 8 9 10
COMMENTS: _____
_____

Movement/Exercise: _____
_____
_____

Energy Level: 1 2 3 4 5 6 7 8 9 10
Stress Level: 1 2 3 4 5 6 7 8 9 10

Notes: (Cravings, Major Breakthroughs, Tough Spots, Symptoms):
_____
_____
_____
_____

"Being an example of health is the best way to motivate others to get healthier. Lead by example"

Day 4
Week 1

Date _____

Breakfast: _____
_____

Lunch: _____
_____

Dinner: _____
_____

Snacks: _____

Sleep:

HOURS: 4 5 6 7 8 9 10   QUALITY: ☺   ☹   ☹

COMMENTS: _____
_____

Movement/Exercise: _____
_____
_____

Energy Level: 1 2 3 4 5 6 7 8 9 10

Stress Level: 1 2 3 4 5 6 7 8 9 10

Notes: (Cravings, Major Breakthroughs, Tough Spots, Symptoms):
_____
_____
_____
_____
_____

"It's not who you are that holds you back, it's who you think you're not."

Day 5
Week 1

Date

Breakfast: _____
_____
_____

Lunch: _____
_____
_____

Dinner: _____
_____
_____

Snacks: _____
_____

Sleep: QUALITY: 😊   😐   🙁

HOURS: 4 5 6 7 8 9 10

COMMENTS: _____
_____

Movement/Exercise: _____
_____
_____

Energy Level: 1 2 3 4 5 6 7 8 9 10

Stress Level: 1 2 3 4 5 6 7 8 9 10

Notes: (Cravings, Major Breakthroughs, Tough Spots, Symptoms)
_____
_____
_____
_____
_____

"A goal is a dream with a deadline."

Day 6
Week 1

Date

Breakfast: _____

_____

_____

Lunch: _____

_____

_____

Dinner: _____

_____

_____

Snacks: _____

_____

Sleep:

QUALITY: ☺ 😐 ☹

HOURS: 4 5 6 7 8 9 10

COMMENTS: _____

_____

Movement/Exercise: _____

_____

_____

Energy Level: 1 2 3 4 5 6 7 8 9 10

Stress Level: 1 2 3 4 5 6 7 8 9 10

Notes: (Cravings, Major Breakthroughs, Tough Spots, Symptoms):

_____

_____

_____

_____

_____

"Nothing is impossible. The word itself says 'I'm possible'"- Audrey Hepburn

Day 7
Week 1

Date _____

Breakfast: _____
_____
_____

Lunch: _____
_____
_____

Dinner: _____
_____
_____

Snacks: _____
_____

Sleep:
HOURS: 4 5 6 7 8 9 10   QUALITY: ☺   😐   ☹
COMMENTS: _____
_____

Movement/Exercise: _____
_____
_____

Energy Level: 1 2 3 4 5 6 7 8 9 10

Stress Level: 1 2 3 4 5 6 7 8 9 10

Notes: (Cravings, Major Breakthroughs, Tough Spots, Symptoms):
_____
_____
_____
_____
_____

"Take care of your body. It's the only place you have to live"- Jim Rohn

WEEK 2

Key achievements from last week:

Symptoms experienced last week:

Goals for the coming week:

Day 8
Week 2

Date _____

Breakfast: _____
_____
_____

Lunch: _____
_____
_____

Dinner: _____
_____
_____

Snacks: _____

Sleep:

QUALITY: ☺   😐   ☹

HOURS: 4 5 6 7 8 9 10

COMMENTS: _____
_____

Movement/Exercise: _____
_____
_____

Energy Level: 1 2 3 4 5 6 7 8 9 10

Stress Level: 1 2 3 4 5 6 7 8 9 10

Notes: (Cravings, Major Breakthroughs, Tough Spots, Symptoms)
_____
_____
_____
_____
_____

"If it doesn't challenge you, it doesn't change you"- Fred Devito

Day 9
Week 2

Date _____

Breakfast: _____
_____
_____

Lunch: _____
_____
_____

Dinner: _____
_____
_____

Snacks: _____
_____

Sleep:

HOURS: 4   5   6   7   8   9   10   QUALITY: 🙂   😐   🙁

COMMENTS: _____
_____

Movement/Exercise: _____
_____
_____

Energy Level: 1   2   3   4   5   6   7   8   9   10

Stress Level: 1   2   3   4   5   6   7   8   9   10

Notes: (Cravings, Major Breakthroughs, Tough Spots, Symptoms):
_____
_____
_____
_____
_____

"It's no coincidence that four of the six letters in health are 'heal'"- Ed Northstrum

Day 10
Week 2

Date [   ]

Breakfast: _____
_____
_____

Lunch: _____
_____
_____

Dinner: _____
_____
_____

Snacks: _____
_____

Sleep: QUALITY: ☺   😐   ☹

HOURS: 4 5 6 7 8 9 10

COMMENTS: _____
_____

Movement/Exercise: _____
_____
_____

Energy Level: 1 2 3 4 5 6 7 8 9 10

Stress Level: 1 2 3 4 5 6 7 8 9 10

Notes: (Cravings, Major Breakthroughs, Tough Spots, Symptoms):
_____
_____
_____
_____

"A positive outlook reinvigorates the mind & soul"- Garnet Hill

Day 11
Week 2

Date

Breakfast: _____
_____
_____

Lunch: _____
_____
_____

Dinner: _____
_____
_____

Snacks: _____
_____

Sleep:
HOURS: 4 5 6 7 8 9 10   QUALITY: ☺   😐   ☹
COMMENTS: _____
_____

Movement/Exercise: _____
_____
_____

Energy Level: 1 2 3 4 5 6 7 8 9 10

Stress Level: 1 2 3 4 5 6 7 8 9 10

Notes: (Cravings, Major Breakthroughs, Tough Spots, Symptoms):
_____
_____
_____
_____
_____

"If you hate starting over, stop quitting!"- Unknown

Day 12
Week 2

Date: _____

Breakfast: _____
_____

Lunch: _____
_____

Dinner: _____
_____

Snacks: _____

Sleep:
HOURS: 4 5 6 7 8 9 10   QUALITY: ☺   😐   ☹

COMMENTS: _____

Movement/Exercise: _____
_____

Energy Level: 1 2 3 4 5 6 7 8 9 10

Stress Level: 1 2 3 4 5 6 7 8 9 10

Notes: (Cravings, Major Breakthroughs, Tough Spots, Symptoms)
_____
_____
_____
_____

"The greatest wealth is health"- Virgil

Day 13
Week 2

Date _____

Breakfast: _____
_____
_____

Lunch: _____
_____
_____

Dinner: _____
_____
_____

Snacks: _____
_____

Sleep:
HOURS: 4   5   6   7   8   9   10   QUALITY: ☺   😐   ☹
COMMENTS: _____
_____

Movement/Exercise: _____
_____
_____

Energy Level: 1   2   3   4   5   6   7   8   9   10

Stress Level: 1   2   3   4   5   6   7   8   9   10

Notes: (Cravings, Major Breakthroughs, Tough Spots, Symptoms):
_____
_____
_____
_____

"It's not about being best, it's about being better than you were yesterday" - Unknown

Day 14
Week 2

Date

Breakfast: _____
_____

Lunch: _____
_____

Dinner: _____
_____

Snacks: _____

Sleep: QUALITY: ☺   ☺   ☹
HOURS: 4 5 6 7 8 9 10
COMMENTS: _____
_____

Movement/Exercise: _____
_____
_____

Energy Level: 1 2 3 4 5 6 7 8 9 10

Stress Level: 1 2 3 4 5 6 7 8 9 10

Notes: (Cravings, Major Breakthroughs, Tough Spots, Symptoms):
_____
_____
_____
_____

"I have decided to be happy because it is good for my health" - Unknown

WEEK 3

Key achievements from last week:

Symptoms experienced last week:

Goals for the coming week:

Day 15
Week 3

Date _____

Breakfast: _____
_____
_____

Lunch: _____
_____
_____

Dinner: _____
_____
_____

Snacks: _____

Sleep: QUALITY: ☺   😐   ☹
HOURS: 4 5 6 7 8 9 10
COMMENTS: _____
_____

Movement/Exercise: _____
_____
_____

Energy Level: 1 2 3 4 5 6 7 8 9 10

Stress Level: 1 2 3 4 5 6 7 8 9 10

Notes: (Cravings, Major Breakthroughs, Tough Spots, Symptoms)
_____
_____
_____
_____
_____

"You are what you eat" - Unknown

Day 16
Week 3

Date: _____

Breakfast: _____
_____
_____

Lunch: _____
_____
_____

Dinner: _____
_____
_____

Snacks: _____
_____

Sleep:

HOURS: 4 5 6 7 8 9 10   QUALITY: ☺   😐   ☹

COMMENTS: _____
_____

Movement/Exercise: _____
_____
_____

Energy Level: 1 2 3 4 5 6 7 8 9 10

Stress Level: 1 2 3 4 5 6 7 8 9 10

Notes: (Cravings, Major Breakthroughs, Tough Spots, Symptoms):
_____
_____
_____
_____

"Being healthy and fit isn't a fad or a trend, it's a lifestyle."

Day 17
Week 3

Date

Breakfast: _____

_____

_____

Lunch: _____

_____

_____

Dinner: _____

_____

_____

Snacks: _____

_____

Sleep:

QUALITY: ☺ 😐 ☹

HOURS: 4 5 6 7 8 9 10

COMMENTS: _____

_____

Movement/Exercise: _____

_____

_____

Energy Level: 1 2 3 4 5 6 7 8 9 10

Stress Level: 1 2 3 4 5 6 7 8 9 10

Notes: (Cravings, Major Breakthroughs, Tough Spots, Symptoms):

_____

_____

_____

_____

"Don't wish for it, work for it"

Day 18
Week 3

Date

Breakfast: _____
_____

Lunch: _____
_____

Dinner: _____
_____

Snacks: _____

Sleep:

HOURS: 4 5 6 7 8 9 10   QUALITY: ☺   😐   ☹

COMMENTS: _____
_____

Movement/Exercise: _____
_____
_____

Energy Level: 1 2 3 4 5 6 7 8 9 10

Stress Level: 1 2 3 4 5 6 7 8 9 10

Notes: (Cravings, Major Breakthroughs, Tough Spots, Symptoms):
_____
_____
_____
_____

"Life is better when you are laughing."

Day 19
Week 3

Date: _____

Breakfast: _____
_____

Lunch: _____
_____

Dinner: _____
_____

Snacks: _____

Sleep:

QUALITY: ☺ 😐 ☹

HOURS: 4 5 6 7 8 9 10

COMMENTS: _____

Movement/Exercise: _____
_____

Energy Level: 1 2 3 4 5 6 7 8 9 10

Stress Level: 1 2 3 4 5 6 7 8 9 10

Notes: (Cravings, Major Breakthroughs, Tough Spots, Symptoms)
_____
_____
_____
_____

"The earlier you start working on something, the earlier you will see results."

Day 20
Week 3

Date _____

Breakfast: _____
_____

Lunch: _____
_____
_____

Dinner: _____
_____
_____

Snacks: _____

Sleep:

HOURS: 4 5 6 7 8 9 10   QUALITY: ☺   ☺   ☹

COMMENTS: _____
_____

Movement/Exercise: _____
_____
_____

Energy Level: 1 2 3 4 5 6 7 8 9 10

Stress Level: 1 2 3 4 5 6 7 8 9 10

Notes: (Cravings, Major Breakthroughs, Tough Spots, Symptoms):
_____
_____
_____
_____
_____

"Always find time for the things that make you happy to be alive"

Day 21
Week 3

Date [ ]

Breakfast: _____
_____
_____

Lunch: _____
_____
_____

Dinner: _____
_____
_____

Snacks: _____
_____

Sleep:
HOURS: 4   5   6   7   8   9   10

QUALITY: 😊   😐   ☹️

COMMENTS: _____
_____

Movement/Exercise: _____
_____
_____

Energy Level: 1   2   3   4   5   6   7   8   9   10

Stress Level: 1   2   3   4   5   6   7   8   9   10

Notes: (Cravings, Major Breakthroughs, Tough Spots, Symptoms):
_____
_____
_____
_____
_____

"Warning: Exercise has been known to cause health and happiness"

WEEK 4

Key achievements from last week:

Symptoms experienced last week:

Goals for the coming week:

Day 22
Week 4

Date _____

Breakfast: _____
_____
_____

Lunch: _____
_____
_____

Dinner: _____
_____
_____

Snacks: _____
_____

Sleep: QUALITY: ☺   😐   ☹
HOURS: 4 5 6 7 8 9 10
COMMENTS: _____
_____

Movement/Exercise: _____
_____
_____

Energy Level: 1 2 3 4 5 6 7 8 9 10

Stress Level: 1 2 3 4 5 6 7 8 9 10

Notes: (Cravings, Major Breakthroughs, Tough Spots, Symptoms)
_____
_____
_____
_____
_____

"People who love to eat are always the best people"- Julia Child

Day 23
Week 4

Date

Breakfast: _____
_____
_____

Lunch: _____
_____
_____

Dinner: _____
_____
_____

Snacks: _____
_____

Sleep:
HOURS: 4 5 6 7 8 9 10   QUALITY: ☺   😐   ☹
COMMENTS: _____
_____

Movement/Exercise: _____
_____
_____

Energy Level: 1 2 3 4 5 6 7 8 9 10

Stress Level: 1 2 3 4 5 6 7 8 9 10

Notes: (Cravings, Major Breakthroughs, Tough Spots, Symptoms):
_____
_____
_____
_____

"We are like a snowflake - all different in our own beautiful way"

Day 24
Week 4

Date

Breakfast: _____
_____
_____

Lunch: _____
_____
_____

Dinner: _____
_____
_____

Snacks: _____
_____

Sleep:

QUALITY: ☺ 😐 ☹

HOURS: 4 5 6 7 8 9 10

COMMENTS: _____
_____

Movement/Exercise: _____
_____
_____

Energy Level: 1 2 3 4 5 6 7 8 9 10

Stress Level: 1 2 3 4 5 6 7 8 9 10

Notes: (Cravings, Major Breakthroughs, Tough Spots, Symptoms):
_____
_____
_____
_____
_____

"Your body is your most priceless possession - you go take care of it!"-Jack Lalanne

Day 25
Week 4

Date

Breakfast: _____
_____

Lunch: _____
_____
_____

Dinner: _____
_____
_____

Snacks: _____

Sleep:

HOURS: 4 5 6 7 8 9 10   QUALITY: :)   :| :(

COMMENTS: _____
_____

Movement/Exercise: _____
_____
_____

Energy Level: 1 2 3 4 5 6 7 8 9 10

Stress Level: 1 2 3 4 5 6 7 8 9 10

Notes: (Cravings, Major Breakthroughs, Tough Spots, Symptoms):
_____
_____
_____
_____
_____

"Today 95% of chronic disease is caused by food choice, toxic ingredients, nutritional
deficiencies and lack of physical exercise!"

Day 26
Week 4

Date

Breakfast: _____
_____
_____

Lunch: _____
_____
_____

Dinner: _____
_____
_____

Snacks: _____

Sleep: QUALITY: ☺   😐   ☹
HOURS: 4 5 6 7 8 9 10
COMMENTS: _____
_____

Movement/Exercise: _____
_____
_____

Energy Level: 1 2 3 4 5 6 7 8 9 10

Stress Level: 1 2 3 4 5 6 7 8 9 10

Notes: (Cravings, Major Breakthroughs, Tough Spots, Symptoms)
_____
_____
_____
_____

"Be the woman (or man) who decided to go for it"

Day 27
Week 4

Date

Breakfast: _____
_____
_____

Lunch: _____
_____
_____

Dinner: _____
_____
_____

Snacks: _____
_____

Sleep:

HOURS: 4 5 6 7 8 9 10   QUALITY: ☺   😐   ☹

COMMENTS: _____
_____

Movement/Exercise: _____
_____
_____

Energy Level: 1 2 3 4 5 6 7 8 9 10

Stress Level: 1 2 3 4 5 6 7 8 9 10

Notes: (Cravings, Major Breakthroughs, Tough Spots, Symptoms):
_____
_____
_____
_____

"A man's health can be judged by which he takes two at a time - pills or the stairs" -Joan Welsh

Day 28
Week 4

Date _____

Breakfast: _____
_____

Lunch: _____
_____
_____

Dinner: _____
_____
_____

Snacks: _____
_____

Sleep:

QUALITY: ☺   😐   ☹

HOURS: 4 5 6 7 8 9 10

COMMENTS: _____
_____

Movement/Exercise: _____
_____
_____

Energy Level: 1 2 3 4 5 6 7 8 9 10

Stress Level: 1 2 3 4 5 6 7 8 9 10

Notes: (Cravings, Major Breakthroughs, Tough Spots, Symptoms):
_____
_____
_____
_____

"Healthy is an outfit that looks different on everybody"

WEEK 5

Key achievements from last week:

Symptoms experienced last week:

Goals for the coming week:

Day 29
Week 5

Date _____

Breakfast: _____
_____
_____

Lunch: _____
_____
_____

Dinner: _____
_____
_____

Snacks: _____
_____

Sleep:

QUALITY: ☺   😐   ☹

HOURS: 4 5 6 7 8 9 10

COMMENTS: _____
_____

Movement/Exercise: _____
_____
_____

Energy Level: 1 2 3 4 5 6 7 8 9 10

Stress Level: 1 2 3 4 5 6 7 8 9 10

Notes: (Cravings, Major Breakthroughs, Tough Spots, Symptoms)
_____
_____
_____
_____

"A person who never made a mistake never tried anything new" -Albert Einstein

Day 30
Week 5

Date: _____

Breakfast: _____
_____

Lunch: _____
_____

Dinner: _____
_____
_____

Snacks: _____
_____

Sleep:

HOURS: 4 5 6 7 8 9 10   QUALITY: ☺   😐   ☹

COMMENTS: _____
_____

Movement/Exercise: _____
_____
_____

Energy Level: 1 2 3 4 5 6 7 8 9 10

Stress Level: 1 2 3 4 5 6 7 8 9 10

Notes: (Cravings, Major Breakthroughs, Tough Spots, Symptoms):
_____
_____
_____
_____
_____

"There is nothing more rare, nor more beautiful than a woman being unapologetically herself" -
Steve Maraboli

30-Day RESULTS

How did it go? Do you feel like it was worth it?

Look back at your symptoms from Week 1. Do you still have all of them? If not, which ones are gone?

Any new symptoms? *(This is perfectly normal - as you become more in tune with your body you'll notice more and more and sometimes even get super nitpicky.)*

Weight is not everything and it might not even be important if you are trying to rid your body of inflammation. Once the body heals, it will "right size" itself. If you are keeping track though, write your starting weight and your 30-day weight in the spaces provided.

Starting Weight _____

Day 30 Weight _____

Congrats! 30 days are done. Now what?

If you've noticed any positive changes over the 30 days, you're probably motivated to continue doing what you've been doing. Especially if a significant number of symptoms have subsided!

If you're interested in using the Paleo (and Autoimmune Paleo and Whole30) diets and lifestyle to continue your journey, I have a lot of resources on my website to help you along the way. Visit thrivingonpaleo.com to learn how I make it work, use Paleo for my autoimmune diseases, and for many delicious recipes.

I also have tons of free Paleo resources, like cookbooks, meal plans, guides for wellness, and so much more in my Paleo Freebie Library. Get the password at thrivingonpaleo.com/freebies

If Paleo isn't your thing, that's ok too! Whatever you choose, seeing tangible changes like reductions in symptoms will help you stick with it. So whether you continue to use this tracker or another one, I hope you continue to see changes in the right direction!

Make sure, whatever you do, that you celebrate each and every win you've achieved over the last 30 days. These small shifts can add up to HUGE results over time, and you should be proud of these!

Shifts like these will serve you for a lifetime.

You deserve lasting health!

Cheering you on,

Michele Spring

Additional Notes

Additional Notes

Additional Notes

Additional Notes

Additional Notes

Made in the USA
Las Vegas, NV
20 August 2021

28450294R00026